Eating GOD'S WAY

CAROLYN JOHANSEN

Carolyn Johansen

WestBow
PRESS®
A DIVISION OF THOMAS NELSON
& ZONDERVAN

Copyright © 2017 Carolyn Johansen.

All rights reserved. No part of this book may be used or reproduced by any means, graphic, electronic, or mechanical, including photocopying, recording, taping or by any information storage retrieval system without the written permission of the author except in the case of brief quotations embodied in critical articles and reviews.

This book is a work of non-fiction. Unless otherwise noted, the author and the publisher make no explicit guarantees as to the accuracy of the information contained in this book and in some cases, names of people and places have been altered to protect their privacy.

Scripture quotations marked NASB are taken from the New American Standard Bible, Copyright 1960, 1962, 1963, 1968, 1971, 1972, 1973, 1975, 1977, 1995 by The Lockman Foundation. Used by permission.

The information, ideas, and suggestions in this book are not intended as a substitute for professional medical advice. Before following any suggestions contained in this book, you should consult your personal physician. Neither the author nor the publisher shall be liable or responsible for any loss or damage allegedly arising as a consequence of your use or application of any information or suggestions in this book.

WestBow Press books may be ordered through booksellers or by contacting:

WestBow Press
A Division of Thomas Nelson & Zondervan
1663 Liberty Drive
Bloomington, IN 47403
www.westbowpress.com
1 (866) 928-1240

Because of the dynamic nature of the Internet, any web addresses or links contained in this book may have changed since publication and may no longer be valid. The views expressed in this work are solely those of the author and do not necessarily reflect the views of the publisher, and the publisher hereby disclaims any responsibility for them.

Any people depicted in stock imagery provided by Thinkstock are models, and such images are being used for illustrative purposes only.
Certain stock imagery © Thinkstock.

ISBN:978-1-5127-8605-7 (sc)
ISBN: 978-1-5127-8603-3 (hc)
ISBN: 978-1-5127-8604-0 (e)

Library of Congress Control Number: 2017907456

Print information available on the last page.

WestBow Press rev. date: 05/11/2017

Contents

Acknowledgments vii

Chapter 1   What Is Eating God's Way All About? 1

Chapter 2   What Went Wrong? 3

Chapter 3   What Does Eating God's Way Not Mean? 11

Chapter 4   What Does the Bible Say? 15

Chapter 5   Why Would I Want to Eat God's Way? 19

Chapter 6   How Do I Know If the Food Is God's? 25

Chapter 7   Does it Cost More? 31

Chapter 8   What Do I Really Need to Eat? 35

Chapter 9   So What Do I Need? 55

Chapter 10   Food as Medicine 59

Chapter 11   Sample Issues That Can Be Helped with Food 69

Chapter 12 What About Supplements?...................................75

Chapter 13 Can't I Ever Have Any Fun?...............................83

Chapter 14 But That's My Favorite Food!............................85

Chapter 15 Fasting...87

Chapter 16 What About the People Around Me? 91

Chapter 17 Your Mouth Isn't the Only Thing That Eats........93

Chapter 18 What Are the Results? 97

Conclusion 99

Acknowledgments

I would like to thank everyone who made this work possible. Most of all, I want to thank my husband who has put up with my years of being in school as well as the time I spent working on all of this. I also want to thank the clients of A Better You. Even though that business no longer exists, it allowed me to have time to study and to fine tune that information into practical helps in the areas of nutrition and weight loss.

Chapter 1

What Is Eating God's Way All About?

> There is a way which seems right to a man,
> but its end is the way of death.
>
> —Proverbs 14:12

Eating God's way is about eating the way God intended man to eat from the beginning of creation. If we look at Genesis, we see that God created a fully functioning world with everything that every living creature needed. Nothing was left out or left to chance.

God first made water. After the air we breathe, water is the most necessary element for life. You can live a long time with little or no food, but you can only live three days without water and only minutes without air.

God had thought all this through when He began creation. God gave us light and darkness because to be truly healthy, all living creatures need both. (Some fish survive in dark caves, but they are few and far between [Genesis 1:3]).

Next, God created plants. Even carnivores need plants to survive. They get their plants by eating animals that eat plants. God had it all figured out (Genesis 1:11).

God created animals after air, water, and plants so that everything that would allow them to survive and thrive was already in place. Nothing was left out or missing (Genesis 1:20–25).

Eating God's way, or doing anything God's way, means going back to the way He designed us to live. It means eating foods in their natural form. This may mean a mostly raw diet, but it doesn't have to. The Bible talks about different ways of cooking, so cooking isn't going against God's plan for us. It means eating foods grown the way God intended. The Bible doesn't talk about factory farms or food processing plants. We need to think about this before we eat food from such places.

CHAPTER 2

WHAT WENT WRONG?

> Enter through the narrow gate; for the gate is wide
> and the way is broad that leads to destruction,
> and there are many who enter through it.
>
> —Matthew 7:13

God made man only after He made everything else so that it was in place for His new creation to thrive. This includes tasks for mankind. We call it the four-letter word *work*! We don't always like doing it, but God knows that without a purpose, mankind won't thrive. He made us for a purpose, and we spend our whole lives looking to fulfill that purpose (Genesis 1:28).

In recent years, mankind has tried to improve on what God has made. God intended the soil to stay rich through a cycle of life, death, and decomposition that returns the nutrients to the earth. Instead, we try to keep our soils strong using chemical fertilizers. Now we don't have to deal with any unpleasant smells coming from the compost piles; we simply put a bag (or ton) of chemicals on our gardens or fields. The plants look fine, so we think we did something good.

We know plants are covered in bugs, which feast on them because even though the plants look fine, they were not all possessing of certain properties that would ward off these pests. God put these pests on earth to clear out weak, dying plants, and they're really doing their jobs!

Man's solution to this situation was to invent pesticides. Now, we just have to spray our plants with another chemical and the bugs will go away. The problem is that each year, we have to use more and more pesticides. We're told that the bugs are adapting, but that would mean the bugs God made are smarter than the men who made the chemicals to get rid of them.

Another problem is that these pesticides kill all the bugs, even the ones we need. God gave each bug a job. Some kill off weak plants. Others clean up after both plants and animals. But there's more to it than that. Some of these flowers produce our food, and some of these bugs pollinate our flowers. If the flowers aren't pollinated, then the plants don't produce any food. Some bugs were put on earth to attack other bugs, and these chemicals are killing off our pollinators as well as the bugs that attack plants.

The next step for man was to make plants with DNA from bacteria, fungi, and even animals that are supposed to fight off the bugs without the help of chemicals. Some of these plants are supposed to make the bugs explode after eating them. A logical question would then be this: Why should these same plants be considered safe for human consumption? I haven't really heard a good answer from the media that keeps telling us that these plants are safe.

What's interesting is that these modifications were supposed to mean a decrease in the need for pesticide and fertilizer use, but sales receipts show that farmers are actually using more to get the same amount of food from the fields.

When farmers were using compost and crop rotation to keep their soils healthy, they grew healthy plants that didn't need a lot of pest control. A small farmer could grow enough food to feed his family, with enough left over to sell or trade for other necessities and even a few luxuries. Now, most big farming corporations in the United States are getting government subsidies so that they can make ends meet.

Farmers are also using more water than ever before. One reason is that with modern irrigation techniques and modern fertilizers, they're growing crops in areas that couldn't support certain plants in the past.

One such crop is cotton. It's being grown in the American Midwest where there are dry prairies, but cotton is a thirsty plant that requires large amounts of fertilizers because these soils aren't rich in the natural nutrients cotton needs. Reports say that this is diminishing underground lakes, which means there won't be enough water to go around. These lakes don't refill every spring like the above-ground ones do. It takes many, many years for the small amount of moisture in these areas to seep through the ground and replenish the underground lakes.

Growing food God's way is more ecologically sound than growing it man's way. You could even say that its good stewardship of the earth God gave us. In the Bible, God talks a lot about being good stewards.

This brief history of our farming practices shows why most of us really don't know what God intended us to eat, and it gets worse from here. People realized that farming wasn't going to make many of them really rich. A peach is just a peach, and you'll buy it from the farmer that's closest to you and who has the best price. That is, until it's made into peach pie. You pay many times more for a peach pie than you would for a peach. When you get several people making peach pies, then you have to figure out a way to make yours taste better and last longer than any other peach pie. So along came the manufacturers and chemists.

By processing our foods, they were able to kill the pesky enzymes that allowed food to spoil quickly. God created these enzymes to help us digest and utilize the nutrients in food. That's okay, though, because the manufacturing process kills those nutrients as well.

As people began eating more and more processed foods, they began expecting food that tasted the same way every time. We expect a brand of orange juice to taste the same no matter what month of the year it's made or how good a growing season the farmer had. To make sure we get what we want, the manufacturers turned once again to the chemists. By purposefully taking the flavor out of our foods and replacing them with chemicals, manufacturers get the same flavor every time.

People praise modern technology for advancements like food safety. You hardly ever hear about people dying from starvation in modernized nations. What you do hear about a lot is people dying from chronic illness. Worse yet are the people who keep living but can't take care of themselves and get no pleasure out of life. Many times they're in constant pain and facing the loss of more and more of their abilities.

Mankind to the rescue once again! We'll just legalize drugs (chemicals) to help these poor, unfortunate people. The problem is that everything in life has side effects. The air we breathe and the water we drink have side effects. They can be good ones or bad ones. Mountain-fresh air has a side effect of being calming and so does the salty ocean air. Smoke-filled air makes it hard to breathe and makes us cough. Water that has been boiled and poured over coffee beans tastes different and gives us energy. Water mixed with artificial colors and flavors tastes good but makes us overly energetic. It has also been shown that, over time, people who drink a lot of this type of water begin to have health problems.

Medications are the same way. We think nothing of taking an over-the-counter painkiller when we have a headache or fever. Parents even give them to their small children. If you read the packages carefully, you will find that each of these medications have side effects that could be dangerous if taken at the wrong time, in the wrong amount, or even for extended periods of time.

Aspirin, the oldest standby, has been shown to cause Reye's syndrome when it's given to small children. Because of this, parents turn to aspirin substitutes like acetaminophen (Tylenol). What they don't know is that, even at the recommended dosage, acetaminophen can cause damage to the kidneys. Sometimes parents give too much or give it too often, compounding the problem.

There's also the problem of multiple over-the-counter medicines that each contain acetaminophen. When given at the same time, or even at overlapping dosages, this can put a child or adult at serious risk.

Everyone seems to realize that senior citizens often take multiple medications. Many times this starts out as a solution to a small problem or they are prescribed something as a preventative measure. When the person has unpleasant side effects (not just the one they were taking it for), they turn again to their doctor. Many doctors then prescribe another medication to take care of the side effects, treating it like a new illness. If they had gotten rid of the first medication, they wouldn't have needed the second one. Over time, the medications begin to pile up. The person may not even know why they're taking them.

God had a different plan. He put plants on earth that will take care of our problems. Sometimes it is the flowers, leaves, stems, or roots of a plant that are most effective. Sometimes it is a combination. Early humans figured out that if you make a tea out of one plant, it helped with one type of discomfort. Sometimes it was a topical application that was needed. Trial and error, and I think, listening to the voice of God guided them into creating a pharmacy of the plants that were available in their area. Different areas had different plants, so there are many available today that can be used interchangeably. We just need to tap into this information that was available to early man but seems to be rapidly forgotten today. Many governments are also trying to outlaw this information. They say it is for our safety, but if it was safe for our ancestors, why would it be unsafe today?

Medicinal plants don't always work as quickly as chemicals. There are situations where we need an answer in a hurry. Once that crisis is over, instead of avoiding plants that "interfere" with a drug, why not look to replace that drug with plants?

Chapter 3

What Does Eating God's Way Not Mean?

> But food will not commend us to God; we are neither
> the worse if we do not eat, nor the better if we do eat.
>
> —1 Corinthians 8:8

Eating more naturally will not make you a more spiritual person, just a healthier one. The Jewish nation was given some dietary rules in the Old Testament. They were told that certain foods were good to eat and certain foods were not. Many of those people thought that God was telling them how to become more spiritual. In reality, God was telling them to be obedient and how to stay healthy. Their spiritual health, like ours, was rooted in how closely they walked with God, not how closely they followed the rules. Following the rules was just an indicator of how closely they were walking with God.

Following the rules in the Bible is different than it used to be. Old Testament believers had a list of rules that were written down. The

Pharisees added to them on a regular basis. When they broke the rules, they were instructed to go to the temple and offer a sacrifice to show that they were repentant of their sins. They believed that if they died between the time they sinned and the giving of that sacrifice that they would die out of favor with God.

With the birth of Christ, everything changed. When Christ started his ministry, he explained that God was offering a New Covenant, a new contract in today's language. He explained that God was offering one sacrifice that would be good for everyone and every sin. It would only have to happen once and never be repeated again. Christ was that sacrifice. His death on the cross was the onetime gift that God gave to all mankind for the forgiveness of their sins. It was for everyone, but only if that person, individually, made the choice to accept that free gift. That acceptance is also a onetime thing. Once we agree that Christ died for our personal sins, and we thank him for that sacrifice there is nothing that can separate us from God.

Many people take that gift as permission to behave in any way they want to. They point out that they cannot lose their salvation through their behavior or what they eat. They are right, but any time we break God's rules there are consequences. They may not be immediate, but they do accumulate over time. There are physical, emotional, and spiritual consequences to our actions.

The spiritual consequences include losing that closeness that we feel with God. Many times it is described as our prayers bouncing off the ceiling. The emotional consequences include losing friendships with the people we hurt through our actions. They can also result in a self-hatred that can lead to personal suffering and addictions to things that make us temporarily forget our problems. These can be alcohol, drugs, and even food. Sometimes we physically hurt ourselves in an attempt to feel better about things, but that doesn't work well either.

The physical consequences can be obvious, but they aren't always. We all know that playing with fire can cause an ugly burn. What many of us don't realize is that eating, drinking, breathing, or applying the wrong things can cause scarring inside our bodies. These scars show up as diabetes, cancer, heart disease, fibromyalgia, ALS, Alzheimer's, and many more of our modern-day illnesses. Eating man's way will not separate you from God, but it might make you meet Him that much sooner, and with a lot less accomplished on this earth.

CHAPTER 4

WHAT DOES THE BIBLE SAY?

> For everything created by God is good, and nothing
> is to be rejected, if it is received with gratitude.
>
> —1 Timothy 4:4

When it comes to eating right, God gave us a head start. He gave the Israelites some rules to go by. What are some of those rules?

Avoid Unclean Foods

Many foods were listed as unclean. If you look carefully at the list of unclean foods, you can see the reasons behind them. Pigs were considered an unclean animal. Modern science has found that pork contains more parasites than any other meat. This is because of the way the pig digests its food and the choices of food the pig makes.

An experiment was done by stacking four pigs in cage, one on top of the other. Only the top pig was fed. The other pigs only got to eat what fell from the top cage. This would include some of the food given to the top pig but also the excrement from that pig. Over time, all four pigs grew and gained weight. The bottom pig did not seem especially different from the top pig, though common sense tells us it got very little of what we would consider food. One might speculate that the bottom pig might have more parasites in its system than the top pig. That information has been deemed less important over time.

Modern pork producers say that pigs are still safe to eat. All you have to do is cook it properly. God knew what he was doing when He told the Israelites to avoid pork. He knew that they did not have stoves and ovens that could be kept at a constant temperature. He also knew that they did not have modern thermometers to ensure that the very middle of the piece of meat had been brought to the right temperature to kill off all of the parasites. For them it was very unsafe to eat that type of meat, so God told them to avoid it. What does that mean today? Modern growing methods are not going to change the anatomy of the animal. The stuff that goes into the animal goes straight into the meat. Modern cooking methods have changed so that meat is not as harmful as it once was. My personal take is that I avoid pork unless it would harm a relationship to do so. And, if a meal at a restaurant comes with a little bit of bacon, I indulge. My body can handle a tiny bit once in a while.

If you look at the other unclean foods in the Bible and compare it to the scientific knowledge we have today, you can find similar stories for each one. Shrimp is listed as an unclean food. I used to love shrimp until it dawned on me that shrimp play the same role underwater that roaches do on land. I would be hard pressed to eat a roach. Its very appearance screams that it is dirty and full of disease. Now I just don't look at shrimp in the same way. Each person must look at the animals they eat carefully to determine for themselves if they are clean. Some people will determine that they will not to eat any animal products.

Eat Clean Foods

Clean foods that are listed in the Bible are now considered mainstream foods. Almost every culture includes them in some way. Even with the clean foods God gave us some rules to follow. One that comes to mind is not cooking a young animal in its mother's milk. This was not a safety issue but more of a moral one. We are to know where our food comes from and have compassion for animals. Cooking a young goat in the milk its mother produced to feed it shows heartlessness toward those animals. Eating animal meat with thankfulness to God and a conviction that the animal led a good life shows compassion.

Early man was not vegetarian. There were times that they ate mostly plant-based foods because animal meat was not in abundance and was not as easily preserved as the plant-based foods. This made meat a luxury item, not a dietary mainstay. The Bible does not call all meat unclean, just certain animals. Modern studies show that the vegetarian diet works well for a while, but in the long term it can cause problems. This fits with the way our ancestors ate during Biblical times.

CAROLYN JOHANSEN

The Bible does not talk about processed foods or genetically modified foods. People during the time the Bible was written would not have understood what God was talking about. This leaves us to look at the effects of these foods on our physical and emotional health to determine if they are what the Bible would refer to as clean or unclean foods.

Chapter 5

Why Would I Want to Eat God's Way?

When you sit down to dine with a ruler, consider
carefully what is before you; and put a knife to your
throat if you are a man of great appetite. Do not
desire his delicacies, for it is deceptive food.

—Proverbs 23:1-3

As mentioned earlier, eating right is not going to make you more spiritual. So why would we want to bother eating differently than the world around us?

God designed us to eat real food. Eating anything else compromises God's plan for our lives. This can be seen in the way we look and feel. People who eat right have a healthy glow about them; they have a bounce to their step. They typically look younger than their age. They can be around sickness without always getting sick. They have energy to do the things they want to do. They don't spend their lives worrying about their aches and pains. They are more attractive to others. They have more pleasant and stable personalities.

People who eat man's way are the opposite. Even with lots of makeup and fancy hair colors, they just look less pleasing. They get sick more often and are sicker when they do. They tend to constantly complain about this or that ache or pain. They have less energy and less enthusiasm for the tasks in front of them. They catch every bug that is going around and even tend to pass it back and forth among household members.

Christians need to be especially aware of this. If someone wants to hear about the joy of following Christ, are they going to ask the person with a smile and a bounce or the one that can barely drag him- or herself from one chair to another? Are they going to believe that you are a new person in Christ when you are always complaining about your latest problem or about the side effects of your latest medication? Think about it from their standpoint. If we are going to ask someone to follow our walk with Christ, we better make that walk look attractive. Man looks at the outward appearance. Shouldn't we be doing everything we can to make that outward appearance something that others would want for themselves?

The healthier we are, the longer we will be on this earth, but more important, the healthier we are, the more energy we will have for the tasks God puts in front of us. When we are eating right we don't need stimulants or pick-me-ups. We also don't spend a lot of time sitting around moping.

People sometimes ask what I did in a day. Frequently, as I list through my tasks I have accomplished, I can see their eyes begin to glaze over. Often they will comment that just hearing about it makes them tired. At other times, when I haven't been eating the way I am supposed to, people will comment that I look tired. On those days I look back on my day and I haven't accomplished nearly as much as I usually do. There is no scientific study that the poor eating has done this for me, but having it happen over and over again convinces me that it is true.

Many people suffer from migraines. I have had several friends that suffered from these horrendous headaches. When they began eating the way God intended and getting the water their bodies need, they have fewer headaches. The ones they did have were much milder. Some of these people went back to their old eating habits, and the headaches came back.

Chronic illness has been linked to lifestyle habits, including eating habits. Diabetes comes in two distinct forms. There is one type where the body doesn't make insulin. This is called Type 1 diabetes. This can either be there at birth or come later in life, usually due to an injury. The normal treatment for this type of diabetes is to replace the missing insulin. The other type of diabetes (Type 2) occurs during the person's life. It is often referred to as insulin resistance. In this form the body quits listening to the insulin the pancreas is making. The word picture that best explains it is this: you hear the doorbell ring and there is no one there when you answer it. Over time you simply ignore the doorbell ringing. In the case of your cells, it is not that there is no blood sugar to welcome into the cell. It is more that the cell is already crammed full and there is no room for more. Sometimes there is room, but the cell has forgotten what the ringing means.

Hypoglycemia is sometimes called prediabetes. With hypoglycemia, the body is extremely efficient in clearing the bloodstream of all blood sugar. This leaves the person with symptoms of low blood sugar. The common treatment for this is to eat something sugary. This quickly brings up the blood sugar levels, but it also triggers the pancreas to produce more insulin, which in turn quickly lowers the blood sugar. It becomes a never-ending dance, which in turn can lead to full-fledged diabetes.

Alzheimer's is sometimes referred to as Type 3 diabetes. This is because many people with Alzheimer's also have a history of hypoglycemia. In addition to hypoglycemia, there are also links to mercury and aluminum in their systems. Mercury and aluminum are not naturally found in our food or water. Mercury comes to us through pollution, dental fillings, and vaccinations. All of these are things that man has added to the way we live. They were not part of God's original design. Aluminum mainly comes through processed foods and cooking our foods in aluminum pans or aluminum foil. It can also come through antiperspirants and other personal care products. High concentrations of aluminum are found in the brains of people who have died of Alzheimer's.

Recently there has been another suggested cause of dementia. This is a disease that in animals is called mad cow disease and in people is called Creutzfeldt-Jakob disease. This disease is spread when animals eat the ground-up body parts of other sick animals. There is a strong suggestion from scientific research that people get it not only through contaminated meat but also contaminated dairy products. Pasteurized dairy products seem to carry more danger of this disease than raw ones. This may be simply because sellers of raw dairy products are much more particular about what the animals eat and the cleanliness of their environment.

These are just a few of the diseases that are strongly linked to diet. Heart disease, fibromyalgia, cancer, autoimmune diseases—all of these and many others are epidemic in our world today, and all of them (and many more) have been linked to a diet high in processed foods. Will eating only a diet of all natural foods guarantee that you won't suffer from any of these diseases? No, there are no such guarantees in life. Not only what you eat today but what you ate yesterday and even what your parents and grandparents ate before you were conceived play an integral part in what diseases you will be susceptible to. Even if we start today by eating only what God has provided for us, we can't undo the past, but it can stop the damage from continuing and give us a better chance at a strong and healthy life.

CHAPTER 6

HOW DO I KNOW IF THE FOOD IS GOD'S?

And in their heart they put God to the test by asking food according to their desire.

—Psalm 78:18

We start our journey into eating God's way by taking an inventory of how we are eating. Nobody likes to keep a food diary, but it is a great way to take a look at what you are putting on your plate, or better yet, in your mouth.

Look over the foods you eat. Did it come from a farm or a factory? Could you buy the ingredients and make it at home in your own kitchen? Can it be put on a shelf and left indefinitely with very little change? Is there an ingredients list with things you don't recognize and can't pronounce? These will help you determine if it is a God made food, or a manmade food. Labeling laws say that the ingredients list should be in the order of the amount of that item in the food. The largest amount is listed first and the least amount is listed last. Manufacturers have gotten around these rules by listing things by multiple names. Sugar is a good example. They use multiple sources for sugar and list each one separately. That makes it look like the amount of sugar is less. Another thing about labeling, all the things in the package don't have to be on the label. Man-made foods are not real foods; they are fake foods, frankenfoods, or food-like substances. Let's look at some examples.

American Cheese Versus Raw Milk Cheese

American cheese slices, boxed cheese, and canned cheese spreads are all man made. Many times there are not even any milk products in them. They are usually made from vegetable oils. They get their color and flavor from chemicals. They can be left on a shelf for a length of time without real changes to them. Many times they will not even mold. They have ingredients lists on the packages that include words that are difficult to pronounce and even more difficult to understand. Raw milk cheese is usually made from milk, rennet, and time. The rennet can be from animal or plant sources. If you were industrious enough you could get rennet yourself, but most cheese makers simply buy it.

Corn Flakes Versus Oats

When have you looked at a field of corn and seen the flakes? That is because corn flakes are not grown, they are manufactured. If you look at the box of corn flakes you will see that there is an ingredient list that contains words that are hard to pronounce.

The box of cereal can sit on the shelf for months without a huge change in appearance. If it has been opened, it might become stale, but it won't turn back into dirt like real food does. Oats on the other hand are real grains. Some of them have been cut, others have been smashed flat. These are ways that man has modified the grains to make them quicker and easier to cook and eat.

Instant oatmeal is more like the corn flakes. If you leave real oats in an opened container on a shelf, it will get bugs and begin decomposing. It doesn't happen quickly, but it does happen. I had a box of instant oatmeal that accidently got put in the garage. The garage had a hole in the back wall and rats got into it. The rats did not touch the instant oatmeal. They would rather eat the cardboard and other things that you would not consider edible.

Once you identify food-like substances in your house, it is time to get rid of them. They fill up the belly, but they don't feed the body. If they aren't in the house it is easier to resist them. Eating God's way takes more time and energy than eating man's way. Just like making a pot of oat porridge with real oats takes more time and energy than mixing a bowl of instant oatmeal, eating God's way means planning ahead and making good choices.

You can buy a loaf of white bread, or you can buy wheat berries and make your own whole wheat bread. The whole wheat sounds like eating God's way until you look at the history of wheat. In the book, *Wheat Belly,* Dr. William Davis looks at the history of the wheat plant. First through hybridization and now through genetic modifications, man has changed the wheat plant drastically. The grain of wheat that you can buy today does not in any way resemble the wheat available in Biblical times. The wheat of today contains a protein that is hard for the human body to digest. This is one reason that more and more people are discovering that they are gluten intolerant. It may not be the gluten but this other protein that they cannot tolerate. Most of the grains available today have the same problem. Man has changed the plant so much that the bread made from it does not resemble the bread mentioned in the Bible. This is one reason I put grains in the same category as sugar and other processed foods.

What did the people in Biblical times eat that is still available today? It was meat, eggs, and dairy from animals that were raised the way God intended. This means that the animals lived in fresh air and sunshine. They found their own foods or were fed foods that they could have found on their own.

Many times the weather is not conducive to cows eating grass year round. It is still eating naturally for those cows to eat the dried grass, which we call hay, during the cold and wet winter months. This is not feeding them unnaturally. Cows on their own will not eat a lot of grains, corn, or soybeans. Feeding them a lot of these would not be natural. In addition, corn and soybeans are two crops that have been heavily genetically modified.

Meat, eggs, and dairy grown God's way have been shown to have more vitamins and minerals than those grown in the CAFO (confined animal feeding operation) method. They also have more of the omega-3 fatty acids (the good ones) and less of the omega-6 fatty acids.

Fruits and vegetables that have been grown organically are the way God intended. Heirloom varieties are even better. These are fruits and vegetables that have been grown the same way for hundreds of years. Fruits and vegetables that have been grown with chemicals contain those chemicals. They also contain fewer vitamins and minerals than their organic counterparts if the organic ones have been grown in good soil. There have been a few studies that cast doubt on the superiority of organically grown foods. When the studies are looked at carefully, it is seen that the foods were grown in poor soil. Part of successful organic gardening is to put back nutrients into the soil through composting and crop rotations.

Herbs and spices can also be a part of eating God's way. Again, you want to get the ones that were grown God's way and not man's way. Eating God's way does not have to be boring. Food cooked (or not cooked) appropriately never has to be boring. You just need to learn a little more about herbs and spices in order to add taste and variety to your meat and vegetables. Poorly prepared natural foods taste bad, no matter how good the original ingredients were. That being said, food grown appropriately will have a lot more natural flavor than food grown chemically. This is why some of the best chefs in the world have their own gardens right outside the back door of their restaurant.

Chapter 7

Does it Cost More?

> For which one of you, when he wants to build a tower, does not first sit down and calculate the cost to see if he has enough to complete it?
>
> —Luke 14:28

Many people think that organic foods cost a lot more than conventional foods. Calorie for calorie, healthy food may cost more, but nutrient for nutrient it is much less expensive. When you start looking at the grocery cart you will see a lot of things in there that have no real food value. Sodas are a good example. They have absolutely no food value, yet they cost money that you could be using for nutrients. Chips and cookies are other examples. So are almost all packaged, processed foods.

When I was first married, the newest rage at the grocery store was prepackaged meals. All the ingredients for the meal were in the box. You just had to add the meat and sometimes some water. I thought it was great until I realized my budget wouldn't stretch that far. By going to the bulk bins I could get the noodles and spices for a lot less money than that box cost. The same is true for any food mix. You may feel like you spend more when cooking from scratch, but the reality is that you are purchasing more for the same amount of money. People don't buy two cups of flour; they buy a five or ten pound bag for the same price or less than that cake mix.

When you only shop the outer edges of the grocery store, you can bring home a lot more nutrition for a lot less money. Think about how your local grocery store is laid out. The produce section is usually toward the front and along one of the outside walls. If you follow that outside wall to the back of the store, you typically run into the meat and dairy sections. Sometimes you will come across the bakery and deli. You can skip those. Fruits and vegetables are not cheap, but they have a lot more nutrition than prepackaged fruit snacks that are mostly sugar.

Buying in bulk is another way of saving money. Grass-fed meats are expensive. If you have a freezer, you can buy meat in bulk and save a lot of money. If you can't afford a whole cow, see if you can split it with someone. Some growers sell quarters or halves. You can even split it down even further with family or friends. Buy fruit and vegetables in bulk as well. Then get into your kitchen and freeze, can, or dehydrate the food to save it for future use.

The money we save by avoiding the junk foods or by avoiding restaurant foods can add up quickly. Then that money can be used for purchasing quality foods and for saving up to purchase in bulk. As you begin eating God's way, you may find you have to spend some of that money for new clothes because you old ones are just too big for you. For most of us, this is a good problem to have!

CHAPTER 8

WHAT DO I REALLY NEED TO EAT?

Then let our appearance be observed in your presence, and the appearance of the youths who are eating the king's choice food; and deal with your servants according to what you see.

—Daniel 1:13

When we think about food, we usually think of filling our stomachs, quenching our thirst, or indulging our taste buds. To truly eat God's way, we need to think about refilling our nutrient bank. If you think of our bodies as having a filing system where each nutrient is stored in a separate drawer, it makes it easier to understand. We are all born with our file drawers prestocked. Some of the drawers are crammed full, and other ones are almost empty or everywhere in between. A couple of the drawers are labeled "toxins." We want those drawers to be empty. Unfortunately, more and more babies are being born with those drawers already containing things, some to the point of overflowing. This is one reason children are getting "adult" illnesses such as cancer and heart disease at a younger and younger age.

What are some of the labels on the other drawers?

Vitamin A

Vitamin A improves eye, lung, skin, hair, teeth, bones, and circulatory health. Deficiency symptoms include many eye disorders; respiratory disorders; and poor skin, hair, nails, and teeth. It can be found in fruits, vegetables, liver, eggs, and milk. In cold weather, or when you consume a lot of vitamin C, your body requires more vitamin A. This is one of the vitamins that you can get too much of. Toxicity symptoms include nausea; vomiting; diarrhea; hair loss; headaches; flaky, itchy, and blotchy skin; blurred vision; and an enlarged liver.

Vitamin B1 (Thiamine),

Thiamin protects against beriberi and aging. It aids in digestion and elimination, stabilizes emotions, and relieves irritability and depression. It helps both the heart and brain. It is found mostly in brewer's yeast, brown rice, organ meats, eggs and nuts. This vitamin is destroyed by cooking, caffeine, alcohol, estrogen and sulfa drugs.

Vitamin B2 (Riboflavin)

This vitamin promotes eye and mouth health as well as healthy hair, skin and nails. Deficiency symptoms include bloodshot eyes, sensitivity to light, itching and burning eyes, cataracts, mouth inflammation, and cracks in the lips and corners of the mouth. It is found mostly in brewer's yeast, blackstrap molasses, organ meats, eggs, and nuts.

Vitamin B3 (Niacin)

This is thought of as a man's vitamin because women need smaller amounts. This vitamin works on the emotions, preventing irritability and depression. It can relieve toothache and backache. The well-known niacin flush improves the skin. It can aid in quitting smoking. It can sometimes relieve Hiatal Hernia (severe heartburn). Vitamin B3 is best found in royal jelly, a product from bees.

Vitamin B-5 (Pantothenic Acid)

This vitamin in involved in all vital functions of the body. It stimulates the adrenal glands, reduces stress, and reduces premature aging. It has also been credited with turning gray hair back to its natural color. It can also correct painful and burning feet, adrenal exhaustion, and emotionally induced asthma. This is another vitamin found in royal jelly and bee pollen.

Vitamin B6 (Pyridoxine)

This one is not as well-known as the other B vitamins. It helps to balance the body's electrolytes, fights anemia, edema (swelling), depression, skin disorders, mouth sores, bad breath, nervousness, eczema, kidney stones, migraines, and senility. One reason we haven't heard of it is that it is found in a lot of foods and supplements are rarely needed. Those foods include brewer's yeast, organ meats, cantaloupe, cabbage, blackstrap molasses, milk, eggs, beef, green leafy vegetables, peanuts, and pecans. It is destroyed through cooking.

Vitamin B12

This is the only vitamin that contains essential mineral elements. It is essential in the production and maintenance of red blood cells, prevents anemia, improves growth, prevents cataracts, improves brain function, and relieves numbness, stiffness, weakness, and soreness in muscles. B12 can be hard for some people to metabolize through digestion. It is offered in shots, time-released pills, and sublingual (melt in the mouth) forms. It is naturally found in milk, eggs, liver, brewer's yeast, peanuts, bananas, sunflower seeds, comfrey leaves, kelp, concord grapes, and bee pollen.

Vitamin B13 (Orotic Acid)

This vitamin is vital for the regenerative processes in cells. It is destroyed by water and sunlight. It can be found in root vegetables and whey.

Vitamin B15 (Pangamic Acid)

B15 is an antioxidant. It helps to prevent oxygen deprivation, extends cell lifespan, regulates fat metabolism, reduces cravings for alcohol, stimulates the nervous system, lowers cholesterol levels, and aids in protein digestion. It is helpful in treating heart disease, angina, and asthma. It is found in whole grains, seeds, nuts, and brown rice. It is destroyed by water and sunlight.

Vitamin B17 (Laetrile)

This is an anticancer nutrient, both for prevention and treatment. It can be found in the seeds of fruits such as apricots and peaches. In high doses (supplement form), it can be deadly, but the amount received from chewing on a seed every day is safe. It helps in reducing high blood pressure, cataracts, and sickle cell anemia. Along with apricot and peach kernels, it is found in cherry and plum kernels, apple seeds, raspberries, cranberries, blackberries, lima beans, mung beans, flax seed, millet, buckwheat, and in kasha and cassava beans.

Vitamin H (Biotin)

It is essential for metabolism of fats and proteins. It keeps hair from turning gray or falling out (going bald). It alleviates eczema, dermatitis, dandruff, seborrhea, skin disorders, lung infections, anemia, loss of appetite, depression, drowsiness, and hallucinations. It is found in brewer's yeast, beef liver, egg yolk, milk, and unpolished (brown) rice. Raw egg whites prevent absorption of this vitamin.

Choline

Although choline is a member of the B vitamin family, it is not known by a number like many of the others. Choline helps us digest and utilize fats and the fat-soluble vitamins. It carries these vitamins across the blood-brain barrier. It also minimizes the buildup of fats in the liver and arteries, and aids them in their job of cleaning the body. It has been found beneficial in preventing and even treating arteriosclerosis, Alzheimer's, high blood pressure, kidney damage, glaucoma, and migraines. It aids in hair growth and baldness prevention. It can be found in egg yolk, liver, and leafy green vegetables.

Folic Acid

We have all heard that folic acid is necessary for the development of the human baby. It also helps in protein metabolism, prevents premature gray hair, and corrects skin disorders. Another unknown function of folic acid is that it reduces pain. Sunlight and vitamin C destroys folic acid. It can be found in leafy green vegetables, organ meats, salmon, milk, carrots, egg yolks, cantaloupe, apricots, pumpkins, and avocados.

Inositol

This is another B vitamin that doesn't go by a number. It nourishes brain cells, lowers cholesterol levels, promotes healthy hair, aids the heart, burns up fat and protects the Myelin sheathing that protects the nerves. Deficiency symptoms include baldness, eczema, eye abnormalities, constipation, and high cholesterol levels. Foods that contain inositol include brewer's yeast, milk, nuts, citrus fruit, and liver.

PABA (Para-aminobenzoic acid)

Although PABA aids metabolism and all vital life processes, it is best seen in its effects to the hair and skin. It can prevent premature graying and reverses graying when taken in quantity. It is also helpful with eczema and lupus. Deficiency symptoms include extreme fatigue, anemia, reproductive disorders, infertility, vertigo, and loss of libido. It can be found in milk, eggs, molasses, and liver. Good bacteria in the gut can synthesis it in the intestines. Eating commercially grown meat, eggs, and dairy and taking antibiotics kill these bacteria.

Vitamin C

People think of vitamin C for colds, but it is also important for the formation of collagen. Collagen is important for the growth and repair of tissue cells, gums, blood vessels, bones, skin, and teeth. It helps the body absorb iron and other nutritional substances. Although vitamin C can be found as a very inexpensive supplement this is not the best form of vitamin C. Foods that contain vitamin C include citrus fruits, rose hips, tomatoes, and green peppers. Be cautious of tomatoes and green peppers because they are nightshades and can increase inflammation.

Vitamin D

We hear a lot about vitamin D these days. More and more studies are showing that this "vitamin" is essential in almost every aspect of our lives. I use the quotes because it isn't like the rest of the vitamin world. This is one that our bodies can manufacture. All we need is some cholesterol and sunlight. (As I am writing this, I can look out the window and watch it snow. Not going to get much sunlight today.)

For those like me that live in a northern climate, work in an office, or can't run around with minimal clothing outside in the sunshine all day, there are other ways to get your vitamin D. Anything that grows in sunlight has a small amount. This would eliminate any fresh foods I can get hold of right now because if they were grown in sunlight they have come a long distance. For most of us, a supplement is the best way to go. Make sure it is a D3, and the best ones contain K2, which helps us absorb it.

Vitamin E

Although this is a fat-soluble vitamin, it is not readily stored in the body. Vitamin E works on other vitamins to get the most effect out of them, both inside and outside of the body. It is among the antioxidants so it helps with slowing down the aging process. It also improves both male and female fertility. When we think vitamin E, most of us think of fish oil, but it can also be found in broccoli, Brussels sprouts, leafy greens, spinach, and eggs.

Vitamin F

This is one you never hear anything about. It is literally the fat vitamin. Unlike what the mass media has been preaching for the last twenty (or more) years, our bodies need fat. Fats provide lubrication for our bodies as well as combining with protein and cholesterol to form new cells.

Sunburn can cause you to become vitamin F deficient. Putting a good quality olive, peanut, coconut, or almond oil on the skin can counteract this.

Vitamin K

This vitamin comes in three forms. If you are looking at supplements, look for K1 or K2, K3 is a synthetic form and not as readily available to the body. Vitamin K is necessary for effective blood clotting. Many times when someone is put on a blood thinner, they restrict vitamin K. Deficiency symptoms include Celiac disease, diarrhea, and colitis symptoms. Good sources of vitamin K include yogurt, alfalfa, egg yolk, kelp, green vegetables, fish oil, and liver oil.

Vitamin P

Many people think of vitamin P as belonging in the vitamin C grouping. The purpose of this vitamin is to increase capillary strength and regulate absorption. This prevents hemorrhaging. This vitamin also prevents high blood pressure, respiratory infection, hemorrhoids, varicose veins, excessive bleeding, eczema, and psoriasis, cirrhosis of the liver, radiation sickness, arteriosclerosis, coronary thrombosis, edema, and inner ear infections. It can be found in the white segments of citrus fruits (pith), strawberries, prunes, apricots, blackberries, cherries, and rose hips.

Vitamin T

Vitamin T helps regulate blood stickiness. This in turn combats anemia and hemophilia. It also improves a fading memory. It can be found in sesame seeds and egg yolks.

Vitamin U

Vitamin U has shown a protectiveness of the lungs. It is thought to help prevent the type of cancer caused by pollutants in the air. It can be found in raw cabbage and sauerkraut as well as in alfalfa.

Along with vitamins, our bodies desperately need minerals. These have been depleted from our soils, so we are having a harder time getting the amounts we need.

Calcium

Calcium is used by the body for many different things. It is found in the bones and teeth as well as in many of the softer tissues of the body. It is essential for proper heart activity as well as blood clotting. It is well-known for reducing insomnia. When you are low on calcium, you can experience muscle cramps, numbness, and tingling in the arms and legs, fragile bones, brittle nails, joint pain, tooth decay, nervousness, depression, irritability, and the symptoms of Parkinson's disease.

Many of us have been taught to drink our milk, but there are much better sources of calcium. These include raw vegetables (especially the dark, leafy ones) sesame seeds, almonds, walnuts, millet, and sunflower seeds. Overdose symptoms for calcium include over calcification of bone joints and kidney tissue. Magnesium can counteract overdose symptoms.

Chlorine

This is not what is found in bleach! That form is harmful. This is one of the natural minerals in salt. It helps the body to clean itself and detoxify. It also combines with hydrogen to produce stomach acid. Deficiency symptoms include impaired digestion, obesity, goiter, underactive adrenals, and meningitis. It can be found in tomatoes, celery, iceberg lettuce, kelp, spinach, cabbage, kale, parsnips, and radishes.

Chromium

This is a necessary mineral that is an important part of many enzymes and hormones. It works with insulin to remove sugar from the blood and into the cells for energy. It also influences how much plaque buildup is in the arteries. We would normally get our chromium through our water, but today's modern water treatment centers have removed it. It can still be found in brewer's yeast and liver. While truly raw sugar contains some, white sugar actually depletes the body of this mineral.

Copper

This mineral is essential to the central nervous system but is also used in the formation of our blood, bone marrow, and muscle tissues. Deficiency symptoms include anemia, loss of hair, trouble breathing, graying of hair, low blood pressure, eczema, enlarged prostate, and sexual indifference. Food that should contain copper, if grown correctly, include leeks; garlic; globe artichokes; parsley; beet root, almonds; green, leafy vegetables; prunes; raisins; pomegranates; and liver.

Fluorine

Many people have never heard of this mineral. They think it means fluoride, which is poisonous to the human body. Fluorine does all the things fluoride has been credited with, including protecting teeth and bones. Deficiency symptoms include tooth decay, failing eyesight, cataracts, falling hair, brittle nails, spongy and bleeding gums, and the symptoms of tuberculosis. It can be found in oats, sunflower seeds, milk, cheese, carrots, garlic, beet tops, green vegetables, and almonds. It is not found in municipal drinking water. That is a different substance.

Germanium

Not the flower! That is a geranium. This is a little known mineral that stimulates the formation of red blood cells. Deficiency symptoms include anemia. It has been shown to reverse some forms of cancer. It can be found in Korean ginseng, garlic, barley, and in the Chinese herbs sanzukon, kashi (not the cereal), and hishi.

Iodine

Iodine is used by the thyroid to make hormones. One of them is throxine. This hormone regulates the body's production of energy and promotes growth and development. Iodine also helps to prevent rough and wrinkled skin and regulates the metabolism, energy production, body weight, and reproductive hormones. Deficiency symptoms include an enlarged thyroid (goiter), lack of intelligence, hair loss, dry skin and hair, anemia, fatigue, loss of sex drive, slow pulse, low blood pressure, weight gain, poor circulation, and estrogen buildup. Prolonged lack of iodine causes thyroid cancer, high cholesterol, and heart disease. Iodine can be found in kelp, dulse, and other seaweeds, as well as Swiss chard, turnip greens, garlic, watercress, pineapple, pears, artichokes, citrus fruit, egg yolks, and seafood.

Iron

We all know iron is important in having healthy blood. Without copper, your body cannot use iron efficiently. It is also necessary in gestation and lactation. It is important in producing myoglobin, which is a substance found in muscle cells and is used in muscle contractions. Most people think of tiredness when there is not enough iron in the body. Other symptoms include pale skin; brittle nails; shortness of breath; depression; a red, inflamed tongue; low blood pressure; dizziness; and lack of interest in sex. A headache on the right side of the head between the eye and the temple is also a sign of low iron. That same headache can be a sign of too much iron. The difference is in what relieves the headache.

If you are low, iron will relieve it; if you are high, zinc will relieve it. Iron can be found in liver, molasses, kelp, yellow dock, beets, and most green vegetables.

Magnesium

New evidence is showing that magnesium, like vitamin D, is involved in many more things than we first thought. It is involved in building strong bones and teeth, muscles, red blood cells, and other soft tissues. Since it is also a catalyst for enzyme reactions almost every function in the body is controlled by magnesium. It has been successfully used to treat heart attacks, nervousness, neuromuscular problems, and depression. Stones (calcification) in kidneys, bladder, or prostate glands can be corrected by taking magnesium. Magnesium can be found in almonds, cashews, dulse, raw and cooked green leafy vegetables, figs, apples, safflower, and sesame. There are estimates that because of magnesium deficiencies in the soil that as much as 80 percent of Americans are magnesium deficient.

Manganese

Manganese is involved in the metabolism of carbohydrates, fats, and proteins. It improves eyesight. Deficiency symptoms include tinnitus (in the left ear), male and female sterility, and loss of muscular strength. It can be found in nuts, beans, egg yolk, and sunflower seeds.

Molybdenum

This little known mineral is involved in the metabolism of carbohydrates and purines. Deficiency symptoms include impotence in older males and esophageal cancer. It can be found in brown rice, millet, buckwheat, brewer's yeast, legumes, and naturally hard water.

Phosphorus

This mineral is the second most abundant mineral in the body. Along with building strong bones and teeth, it is essential in having a healthy brain and nerves. Deficiency symptoms include rickets, insanity, memory loss, failing eyesight (left eye), loss of hair, cataracts, rheumatism, neuralgia, tooth decay, spongy and bleeding gums, and tuberculosis. It can be found in rice bran, wheat bran, pumpkin and squash seeds, wheat germ, sunflower seeds, brazil nuts, and safflower seeds. Sugar destroys phosphorus in the body.

Potassium

Potassium controls the water kept inside the cells. It must be in the appropriate ratio with sodium to prevent either heart attacks or strokes. If the potassium level is too low compared to sodium, the body will retain water.

You can tell if your ratio is out of balance if you have symptoms of Bell's palsy. If it is on the right side it shows a potassium deficiency and if it is on the left side it shows a sodium deficiency. Sometimes these signs can be seen in the way people frown.

High blood pressure (diastolic or lower number) can be reduced with potassium. Although many people who have heart problems are cautioned to reduce their sodium intake increasing their potassium intake can do more good. Potassium can be found in potatoes, oranges, tomatoes, bananas, dulse, kelp, parsley, apricots, and dates.

Selenium

Selenium is a mineral antioxidant. Selenium protects against free radical damage, mercury poisoning, and liver damage. It is utilized by the male reproductive system in the manufacture of semen. For women it can alleviate hot flashes and other menopausal symptoms. Deficiency symptoms include liver damage, muscle degeneration, premature aging, heart disease, and muscular dystrophy. It has also been linked to the development of cancer, especially in the gastrointestinal tract. This is one mineral that you can get too much of in your body. Overdose symptoms include loss of hair, brittle fingernails, irritability, and a degeneration of the spinal cord, which can result in paralysis. Selenium can be found in onions, milk, eggs, kelp, garlic, mushrooms, organically grown produce, seafood, and brewer's yeast.

Silicon

Silicon is used by the body in connective tissues, bones, teeth, hair, and nails. A silicon deficiency can be mistaken for epilepsy. Other symptoms include wrinkles, loss of hair, poor bone and teeth development, insomnia, osteoporosis, carbuncles, boils, abscesses, chronic fatigue, memory problems, and nervous disorders. It can be found in young green plants, horsetail, alfalfa, nettles, kelp, bamboo, flaxseed, apples, strawberries, grapes, beets, onions, parsnips, almonds, peanuts, and sunflower seeds.

Sodium

Sodium is a key element for the body. As mentioned in the potassium section an imbalance between the two where sodium is low can cause a stroke on the left side of the body. In addition to balancing potassium, sodium is used in the formation of saliva and digestive enzymes. Sodium balances calcium and magnesium and helps the body to utilize them properly. Many doctors recommend a low sodium diet. What accomplishes the same thing without the risk of Bell's palsy or stroke is to balance sodium and potassium. Signs that you need more sodium include perspiring more, dry and chapped lips, constipation, diarrhea and gas, high systolic blood pressure, nausea, muscular weakness, heat exhaustion, mental apathy and respiratory failure. Increased arthritis pains or sciatica pain on the left side of the body are signs of sodium deficiency as well as numbness in the foot and toes. Long-term sodium deficiency can lead to Type 2 diabetes. Celery is one of the best sources for nutritional sodium as well as carrots, kelp, Irish moss, olives, and dulse.

Sulfur

Sulfur is known as the beauty mineral because it is found in abundance in skin, hair, and nails. It aids in dissolving acids in the body, improves circulation, and normalizes heart action. It also increases bile function, thus cleaning the digestive tract. It is necessary for the formation of collagen, which prevents aging. Deficiency symptoms include eczema, constipation, phlegm, exhaustion, and a drop in voice pitch. Sulfur can be found in garlic, onions, radishes, turnips, horseradish, kale, watercress, cabbage, cranberries, and eggs.

Zinc

Zinc is found throughout the body. It is essential for the hormonal system, especially the prostate gland. It increases wound healing and normalizes insulin levels as well as reducing cholesterol levels. Deficiency symptoms include slow growth, birth defects, underdeveloped sex organs, enlargement of the prostate gland, impaired sexual functioning, infertility, slow healing of wounds, frequent infections, and skin diseases. White spots on finger and toe nails as well as a loss of taste and smell are common. Zinc can be found in lean beef, beef liver, pumpkin seeds, sunflower seeds, Brazil nuts, cashews, tuna, and peanuts.

Many people can balance their nutritional needs simply by eating a wide variety of foods and concentrating on the ones that give the most nutrients for the calorie content. Others need to look at specific deficiency symptoms and increase the foods that contain the nutrients listed with the deficiencies. If the deficiencies are really bad, you may want to consider supplementing for a while until those symptoms decrease or go away. Always use caution when supplementing. Make sure your supplements are all natural and look for new symptoms that indicate another nutrient that is becoming unbalanced.

Chapter 9

So What Do I Need?

> Then God said, "Behold, I have given you every plant yielding seed that is on the surface of all the earth, and every tree which has fruit yielding seed; it shall be food for you."
>
> —Genesis 1:29

What you need is very individualized. Everyone needs a certain amount of the basics. We all need a well-rounded diet that is full of nutrition. We all need to avoid foods that lack nutrition. A good way of thinking of this is to think of a rainbow.

A rainbow has many different colors in it. Food comes in all those colors as well. In foods, the different colors show that the food contains different nutrients. Red and orange colored foods (naturally colored) show that the food is high in vitamin C and other antioxidants. Red can also indicate the presence of lycopene. Yellow indicates manganese. Green vegetables, in general, have vitamin A. Blue foods indicate antioxidants. Eating a variety of colors (thence the rainbow) at each meal ensures you are getting a variety of nutrients. This does not ensure you are getting everything you specifically need, but it does mean you are getting a broad variety. This approach is similar to taking a multivitamin. It says you are getting a wide variety. If you have specific needs, you will need to address those needs in addition to eating a rainbow diet.

Back in the 1800s, and even before then, man noticed that lacking certain nutrients caused certain illnesses. Rickets and beriberi come to mind. As scientific research has improved, other connections are being made. One of the most recent ones is Alzheimer's. There is strong evidence that this illness is caused by a combination of deficiencies and toxicities. The toxicities include aluminum, which is leeched from cooking utensils and absorbed through antiperspirants. But there is more to it than just the toxicities.

New evidence shows that we can be deficient in fats. For a long time, we were taught to avoid all fats or to only consume fats that came from vegetables. Now we find that those vegetable fats are not good for us. When you think of corn, do you salivate over the oil in it? No, because the only way to get the oil out of corn (and most other vegetables) is to use high heat and chemicals. The heat turns the oil rancid, and the chemicals stay in the oil. These oils are not good for our bodies. Our bodies use saturated fats to repair and replace brain and nerve cells. If someone is deficient in good fats in their bodies, they will have a harder time repairing the damage.

As mentioned previously, Alzheimer's is starting to be known as Type 3 diabetes. A lack of fats and the increase of carbohydrates seem to play a big part in developing this disease.

CHAPTER 10

FOOD AS MEDICINE

*No longer drink water exclusively, but use a little wine for
the sake of your stomach and your frequent ailments.*

—1 Timothy 5:23

Many people think only crazy people would use everyday foods as medicine, but let's think about this a minute. Man survived many generations between the time of Adam and Eve and the introduction of modern medicine with its surgeries and chemicals. Some of the early "medicine" was indeed crazy, but not everyone died at a young age. How did those people survive and even thrive? Many of them identified foods that were helpful in many different situations.

These days we lump some of them into the term *herbs*, but they do not all fall into the dictionary definition of that term. These were plants that were found to be helpful.

A good example of this is white willow bark. This is the bark of the white willow tree. A tree is not by definition an herb, but this bark is useful! Scientific analysis shows it to be almost the same as aspirin. In fact, many believe that it is the natural substance that prompted the chemical compound that we call aspirin. Just like its chemical copy, white willow is useful in reducing pain, swelling, and inflammation. It is also useful in relaxing a person, allowing them to get the healing rest they need. In addition to all of this, it boosts the immune system, allowing it to work better and heal the person faster.

Our ancestors did not have antibiotic ointments to put on their cuts and scrapes. Yes, many people died of minor injuries that became infected, but many people did not. The difference was those that healed were aware of keeping the wound clean. They used substances like olive oil to kill the germs. The story of the Good Samaritan (Luke 10:30-37) talks of him putting oil on the man's wounds. This was to kill the germs and help keep the dirt out. They also used wine, peppermint, thyme, myrrh, garlic, and honey. We still have these things today. With the advent of "super bugs," these old-fashioned remedies are proving to be more powerful than the chemical antibiotics.

Many people know about the wonderful healing properties of aloe vera, when the slimy inner gel of the leaves is used topically. What they are not aware of is that the same plant can be used internally to heal the body. It has been shown useful in healing cuts, bruises, ulcers, soft tissue injuries, and even arthritis. Internally, aloe can be taken as a liquid or as capsules that contain the gel or a powdered version of the gel. It has also been shown to be useful in cases of high blood pressure, multiple sclerosis, stomach ulcers, hair loss, infected gums, shingles, burns, allergies, and many autoimmune problems. These all sound unbelievable, but when you realize that the natural compounds in the aloe plant stimulate the human immune system to work better you can see that any issue in which a strong immune system can speed healing would be helped by this plant.

Almonds are another common food that have medicinal uses. The nut we commonly think of as almonds are technically sweet almonds. Bitter almonds contain a lot of cyanide, which is poisonous. Almond gruel was used for centuries for abdominal or intestinal pains. They were also used for any of the "stone" ailments, such as those of the kidneys, bladders, and biliary (bile or gallbladder) ducts. Mixed with things such as lard, bee's wax, and onion juice, almond oil make a very effective anti-wrinkle cream. Eating almonds also reduces cholesterol and strengthens the heart. Even the bitter almond has been found somewhat useful in battling cancer.

Parsley is considered a cleansing herb. It stimulates the body to release fluids, allowing them to leave the body in the form of urine. Because of this, it has been successfully used to cleanse and heal the kidneys as well as joints. This is true because parsley contains high amounts of vitamin A and vitamin C, as well as iron. Vitamin A deficiency has been linked to hernias.

Parsley is also famous for neutralizing odors, such as alcohol or garlic. This is because it contains large amounts of chlorophyll. It also helps prevent indigestion. Because of its cleansing power, it should not be eaten in large amounts by pregnant women or nursing mothers. It can cause the uterus to contract, causing miscarriage.

Mint covers a whole family of plants. All of them seem to have some type of therapeutic usage. Which one you choose, and how you want to use it, will depend on the ailment. Mint plants have been credited for helping with influenza, herpes, mumps, streptococcus aureus (strep), candidas (yeast infection), muscle spasms, digestion problems, nausea, colic, irritable bowel syndrome, gallstones, arthritis, headaches, toothache, mental decline, abdominal pains and cramps, lack of menstruation, insomnia, shingles, cold sores, burns, wounds, colds, sinus infections, bronchitis, and emphysema.

Peppermint (and almost any plant in the mint family) is good for numerous issues. It works on some things just by breathing in the pleasant aroma of the plant. Other times it is recommended to drink a tea made from its leaves or apply it directly to the skin. It has been recommended for abdominal cramps, arthritis, bronchitis, burns, colds, flu, sinus problems, cold sores, digestive problems, emphysema, gallstones, headaches, insomnia, irritable bowel syndrome, menstrual cramps, senility, shingles, and toothaches. It sounds like one of those foods you don't ever want to be without!

Rosemary is part of the mint family. It has been used to fight cataracts, heart palpitations, hair loss, lack of energy, and mental decline. It has also been used in the treatment of hyperthyroidism. Rosemary is known for helping with cataracts, hair loss, heart palpitations, memory problems, and to increase energy.

Wine is well known as a way to beat stress, but the resveratrol in it is highly recommended for the heart. It is also a very powerful antioxidant. It can be used as an antiseptic. Evidence shows that it reduces angina pain. It has been effective against genital warts, and hepatitis.

Sage is a spice that is much more powerful than we think. It is useful in preventing mental decline, bleeding gums, excessive bleeding, diabetes, fever, stimulation of hair growth, reduction in intestinal spasms, in fighting kidney infections and liver problems, and in soothing laryngitis and tonsillitis. In extremely high doses, sage may cause convulsions, so use it wisely.

Walnuts taste good and are a great source of proteins, fats, and fiber. They are frequently combined with apples and used for treating gallstones and kidney stones, an underactive thyroid, and skin problems such as warts, acne, age spots, and psoriasis. Because walnuts contain a lot of omega-3 fatty acids, they reduce inflammation. They have also been known to reduce cholesterol levels and prevent heart attacks. Walnuts are known to stimulate brain cells and enable clearer thinking.

Some people avoid garlic because of its strong taste and smell. But it is one of the most useful foods God has given us. Since biblical times, it has been used to kill bacteria and viruses in both the human body and the air around us. It has been used to relieve the pain of a toothache. King Solomon recommended it for epileptic seizures.

It is known as a sedative and tranquilizer. It has been used to treat asthma and bloody coughs, such as found in tuberculosis. It cuts phlegm, fights infections, and clears sinuses, bronchial tubes, and lungs. It has been said to kill leprosy, gonorrhea, and gangrene.

It doesn't even have to be eaten to be effective. A garlic plaster or even just a clove of garlic rubbed on the feet can reduce coughing. Putting it on the feet has also been shown to be an effective cure for nosebleeds as well as convulsions. Before antibiotics, it was used to fight streptococcus, salmonella, dysentery, eye infections, typhoid, cholera, and tuberculosis. It can prevent blood clots. It has been known to relieve asthma, bronchitis, emphysema, and a host of other respiratory ailments. The use for garlic goes on and on. We haven't even begun to scratch the surface here.

Another food that is a lot more pleasant tasting and smelling are grapes. It is not a coincidence that wine was made from grapes during biblical times. Now we know that wine can be made from just about any fruit, but back then, wine meant grapes. In biblical times, wine was used as a disinfectant, an anesthetic, a pain reliever, a sleep aid, and used to improve digestion, strengthen weak hearts, and improve breathing.

We have always thought it was the alcohol content in wine that made it a great disinfectant, but even without the alcohol wine is as effective (or more so) as penicillin. What's more, wine can kill viruses as well. It has been shown to be effective against polio, herpes, meningitis, hepatitis, cholera, and influenza. It has even been shown to fight heart disease and cholesterol. This does not give us permission to get drunk. With excess the benefits diminish and the risk of cancer increases exponentially.

Grape seed extracts have been found to be antioxidants that are more powerful than vitamin C. These have proven to be valuable in any of the vein disorders, including varicose veins, diabetic retinothapy, and macular degeneration. Grapes themselves have been shown to be as valuable as hormone replacement therapy in the treatment of osteoporosis. They have been used to dissolve growths and fibrous tissues. Diseased tissues such as ulcers, abscesses, and fatty degenerations have been shown to dissolve and be taken from the body through natural elimination channels.

We have all heard glowing reports from the use of apple cider vinegar. Part of the reason is that apples are high in potassium, which seems to be lacking in our modern food supply. Made into vinegar, it is extremely antibacterial. It also dissolves deposits in your system that causes many of your aches and pains. These include hardening of the arteries and deposits in the kidneys and bladder that cause inflammation. It has also proven helpful with allergy symptoms, such as itchy and watery eyes, runny nose, postnasal drip, sinus infections, and congested sinuses. Many women swear by apple cider baths or douches for pain and itching in the vagina. It has been shown to strengthen muscles and melt away fat. This is great for someone wanting to lose weight. It could also be helpful for someone with a muscle wasting disease such as multiple sclerosis.

Cabbage is a common, everyday food. It has been found to be helpful in asthma, ulcers, osteoporosis, edema (retaining water), arthritis, boils, eczema, infected wounds, nervous disorders, bladder problems, shingles, cold sores, acne, syphilis, hemorrhoids, sciatica, dental pain, gout, colic, headaches, respiratory illnesses, and animal bites. That's a lot of usefulness for the plain old cabbage.

Cantaloupe is believed to prevent heart disease and stroke.

Along with relieving gout, celery has also been shown to be helpful with heart arrhythmias, blood pressure, and cholesterol. Celery juice has also been credited with preventing and even reversing cataracts.

Cinnamon is a very powerful antiseptic. It kills bacteria such as botulism and staph. The juice of the leaves of a cinnamon plant has been shown to kill the germs that cause tuberculosis. Because of this antibacterial effect, it has been shown to be helpful with urinary tract infections.

Honey is a very valuable healing tool. In biblical times, it was known to treat arthritis, asthma, burns, constipation, hay fever, hemorrhoids, migraines, shingles, ulcers, and battle wounds. In modern times, honey has been proven to be a better antibiotic than penicillin. Therefore, it could be useful with typhoid, bronchitis, pneumonia, peritonitis, and dysentery, as well as any other sickness truly caused by germs. It has been known to relieve pain, kill gangrene, soothe chickenpox, treat boils, and heal burns. It has been used for respiratory problems such as asthma and hay fever. Although it is a sugar, honey has been used successfully as part of a treatment for diabetes. There is even evidence that honey can be helpful with stomach ulcers and headaches; even migraines. Ironically, because of its pain relief it has been used for things such as bee and hornet stings. Evidence shows that once again these are just the tip of the iceberg.

The list of things that olive oil is used for is a page long. It is thought that it is the omega-3 fatty acids in the olive oil that make it such a universal cure all. If you combine it with other foods high in omega-3 fatty acids such as flax, grass fed butter, lard, and meat and free range eggs you would go a long way to inducing good health.

Many people don't think of parsley as a food, but it can be as such. Used in different ways, it can be helpful with allergies, diabetes, used as a diuretic, assist with hernias, menopause symptoms, prostrate issues, and psoriasis.

Even the humble radish has some medicinal purposes. It (or its oil) has been used for cancer and gallstones.

These are just a few common foods that have been found to be helpful with many different health issues of the human body. They are examples to show that God provided remedies to every illness from the time He created the earth.

God made whole foods. While man tries to find the "active ingredient" and synthesize that to make a drug, it will never be as effective as the whole food. The "other" ingredients were not included haphazardly. God put them there to either enhance or protect us from the "active ingredient."

Eating a wide variety of foods will ensure good overall health. Remember, I said *foods*. This does not include anything that came from a factory or was created or raised in a way different than God intended. If you already have a health problem, you will need to research that and determine what combination of real foods will give you the best fighting chance. Sometimes our deficiencies are so great that we need to use supplements for a while. Supplements, the truly good ones, are simply concentrated whole foods.

Many foods show what they are good for by their shape. Walnuts look like the two halves of the brain, and are known to improve the brain. Avocados are shaped like a uterus, and are recommended for female issues. Figs look like the male reproductive organs.

Next time you are around your favorite produce, let your imagination run wild as to what the different vegetables look like. Then do a little research. You may be pleasantly surprised!

Chapter 11

Sample Issues That Can Be Helped with Food

Bless the Lord, o my soul, and forget none of His benefits;
who pardons all your iniquities; who heals all your diseases.

—Psalm 103:2–3

Arthritis is a toxicity disease that causes the joints to become inflamed and painful. It is usually looked at as an autoimmune disease, but it is because of toxicities in the body that the immune system goes into overdrive and begins fighting the body. Arthritis is painful and eventually robs a person of their mobility. Foods that either help the body to release the toxins, reduce the pain and inflammation, or adjust the immune system to where it is working correctly include aloe vera, cabbage, cod liver oil, dandelion, garlic, ginger, nettle, peppermint, and wheatgrass juice.

Asthma is a condition where it is difficult to get a full breath. Foods that have been found helpful include cabbage, elderflower tea, garlic, honey, juniper berries, lavender, mustard, nettle, omega-3 fatty acids, and thyme. The same list of foods is helpful with bronchitis; by association we can assume they would be helpful with any case of chronic obstructive pulmonary disease (COPD), no matter what the source.

Emphysema is an illness that causes the person to have trouble breathing. It is one of the illnesses that now go under the heading of COPD. Besides lifestyle changes such as getting away from all types of air pollution, including smoking, perfumes, and air fresheners, there are some foods that help open the airways. These include garlic, juniper berries, any food high in omega-3's, peppermint, and wheatgrass juice.

A good emergency beverage that will temporarily open constricted airways is coffee. Coffee has been recommended for those having an asthma attack and are unable to find their inhaler.

We all get colds from time to time. The foods to concentrate on include elderflower tea, garlic, juniper berries, lavender, mustard (the plant, not the condiment), olive oil, peppermint, and thyme.

Diabetes is epidemic in our world today. As we discussed in chapter 5, there are two types of diabetes. Type 1 cannot be easily reversed, but type 2 can. If a person quits eating all sugars and grains and concentrates on eating low-glycemic (low sugar) vegetables, meats, and fats, they can lower the amount of insulin the body produces and wake up the muscles to utilize the insulin appropriately. Foods that help with this process include dandelion, garlic, olive oil, parsley, cinnamon, and any food high in omega-3 fatty acids.

Gallstones are typically calcium or calcium-like stones that build up in the gallbladder. They have been blamed on too much uric acid in the body but are more commonly caused by too little pure water. Foods that help with gallstones include chamomile tea, chicory, dandelion tea, grapes, peppermint, and radishes.

Gout is another painful problem that is blamed on too much uric acid. The body produces uric acid when it does not digest proteins completely. A hundred years ago, only the very rich complained of gout. They were the only ones that could afford an overabundance of protein-rich foods. Foods that counteract gout include cabbage, celery, chicory root, mustard, nettle, thyme and watercress. The best way to prevent and recover from a case of gout is to ensure that you are completely digesting your foods. Enzymes are the key. Protease is the enzyme that is specifically known for digesting proteins.

High blood pressure is a common ailment today. There are multiple causes which include stress, dehydration, an imbalance between sodium and potassium, and narrowing of the arteries due to plaque buildup. Foods that help lower blood pressure include aloe vera, celery, garlic, hawthorn berry, honey, nettle, olive oil, and other omega-3-rich foods. Hawthorn berry is also useful with low blood pressure as it tends to normalize either extreme.

Shingles are a side effect of chickenpox that occurs later in life. The virus that causes chickenpox is extremely hard to kill and has the ability to go dormant when under attack. Later, when the immune system is low, it revives and produces shingles. These are very painful blisters that can occur anywhere on the body. Foods that help combat shingles include aloe vera, cabbage, peppermint, watercress, and wheat germ oil. Anything that soothes the pain and boosts the immune system will be helpful during an attack.

Many people suffer from diverse stomach problems. Depending on the cause, aloe vera, almonds, barley, cabbage, chamomile, dandelion, grapes, olive oil, and thyme can be helpful.

Toothaches typically send us to the dentist, but if you have to wait for an appointment you might try cloves, aloe vera, garlic, olive oil, peppermint, or thyme to temporarily soothe the ache.

Ulcers can be in the stomach; this term is also used for other sores on the body. Foods that are helpful include aloe vera, cabbage, chamomile, essiac tea, honey, and walnuts.

Weight loss is a popular topic. Besides cutting out the sugars and starches and increasing your exercise, other natural weight-loss aids include apple cider vinegar, celery, dandelion, elderberries, and wheatgrass juice.

Alzheimer's disease attacks the brain and robs its victims first of their short-term memories, then their cognitive abilities. Over time they lose their long-term memories and finally their autonomic functioning, which leads to death. Foods that slow and sometimes reverse this disease include coconut oil, rosemary, and sage.

Cataracts are like having sunglasses inside the eyes that you can't remove when you come indoors. If bad enough cataracts can reduce the light from entering the eye enough to cause blindness. The modern solution is to surgically remove them. People have been able to postpone or avoid surgery consuming celery, grapes, honey, and rosemary.

Cholesterol is considered dangerous in our world today. In truth, it is an indicator of the overall inflammation of the body. Reducing the inflammation will reduce the cholesterol. Reducing or eliminating sugars and grains goes a long way to reducing inflammation.

These are just some examples of ways that you can improve your health by what you eat. For your particular issues consider seeing a naturopath to help guide you.

CHAPTER 12

WHAT ABOUT SUPPLEMENTS?

> Then God said, "Behold, I have given you every plant yielding seed that is on the surface of all the earth, and every tree which has fruit yielding seed; it shall be food for you;
>
> --Genesis 1:29

There are times we cannot eat enough of the foods we need to replenish our bodies in a timely manner. This is where supplements come into play. A good supplement is simply a concentrated form of food. Supplements that are not natural do not do the body any good, and, in fact, can make the deficiencies worse. One way to tell if a supplement is natural is to look at its size. Real food can only be concentrated down so far, so high-quality supplements tend to be large capsules with directions to take more than one of at a time. Synthetic or chemical vitamins tend to be small. If the bottle contains tiny little pills and says you only need to take one to get all the nutrients you need, you can bet they are full of chemicals and not foods. Another way to determine if your vitamin is food or chemical is to look at the ingredient list. Natural ingredient's scientific names start with a D while chemical ones start with an L.

If supplements are concentrated foods, then essential oils are concentrated supplements. Essential oils are typically around a hundred times more potent than the plant they are made from. Because of this, they have a much stronger influence on the human body than the foods themselves. Most essential oils are used either by breathing them in (referred to as aromatically) or by diluting them and putting them on the skin (referred to as topically). There are a few than can be ingested, but use extreme caution when doing this. Essential oils are categorized by what they do for the body as well as the elements present in them. They are said to contain such things as terpenes, camphene, alcohols, esters, aldehydes, ketones, phenols, thymol, and oxides. Each of these has a different influence on the human body. The study of essential oils can be fascinating. Here are some sample uses for essential oils.

Basil essential oil is known for its combination of alcohols, esters and oxides. It is considered an antibacterial, anti-infectious, anti-inflammatory, antioxidant, antispasmodic, antiviral, and has been used as a decongestant, diuretic, disinfectant, and stimulant. Historically, it has been used for respiratory problems, digestive and kidney ailments, epilepsy, insect or snake bites, fevers epidemics, malaria, migraines, liver and gallbladder problems, mental fatigue, and menstrual problems. It can be used aromatically, topically, and orally.

Black pepper essential oil is known for its combination of terpenes, oxides, and aldehydes. It is considered an analgesic, anticatarrhal, anti-inflammatory, antiseptic, antispasmodic, antitoxic, and used as an expectorant, laxative, and stimulant. Historically, it has been used for treatment of malaria, cholera, and digestive problems. It can be used aromatically, topically, and orally.

Cilantro essential oil is known for its aldehydes, alcohols, and phenols. It is considered antibacterial. Historically, it has been used for anxiety and insomnia. It can be used topically or orally. It should be used with caution on young children.

Clove essential oil is known for its phenols, oxides, and ketones. It is considered to be an analgesic, antibacterial, antifungal, anti-infectious, anti-inflammatory, antiparasitic, antiseptic, anti-tumor, antiviral, disinfectant, antioxidant, and immune stimulant. Historically, it has been used for skin infections, digestive upsets, intestinal parasites, toothaches, diarrhea, hernia, bad breath, bronchitis, impotence, intestinal parasites, memory deficiencies, pain, and infected wounds. It can be used aromatically, topically, and orally. Repeated topical use can cause skin sensitivity.

Eucalyptus essential oil is known for its oxides, terpenes, alcohols, and aldehydes. It is considered to be an analgesic, antibacterial, anti-catarrhal, anti-infectious, anti-inflammatory, antiviral, insecticidal, and expectorant. Historically, it has been used for treatment of arterial vasodilation, asthma, brain-blood flow, bronchitis, congestion, cooling, coughs, diabetes, disinfectant, dysentery, ear inflammation, emphysema, fever, flu, hypoglycemia, inflammation, eye inflammation, kidney stones, lice, measles, neuralgia, neuritis, sore muscles, pneumonia, respiratory viruses, shingles, sinusitis, and tuberculosis, and has been used as an expectorant. It can be used aromatically and topically.

Frankincense (yes, what the wise men brought Mary and Joseph) essential oil is known for its terpenes and alcohols. It is considered an anti-catarrhal, anticancer, antidepressant, anti-infectious, anti-inflammatory, antiseptic, anti-tumor, and used as an expectorant, immune stimulant, and sedative. Historically, it has been used for Alzheimer's, arthritis, asthma, balance, aging, brain injury, breathing, cancer, coma, concussion, confusion, coughs, depression, fibroids, genital warts, hepatitis, immunity boosting, vision, infected wounds, inflammation, liver, memory, mental fatigue, warts, wrinkles, and ulcers. It can be used aromatically, topically, and orally.

Ginger essential oil is known for its terpenes, alcohols, ketones, and aldehydes. It is considered antiseptic and has been used as a laxative, stimulant, tonic, and making a person warm. Historically, it has been used to treat angina, diarrhea, gas, indigestion, low libido, morning sickness, nausea, rheumatoid arthritis, scurvy, vertigo, and vomiting. It can be used aromatically, topically, and orally. Repeated topical use can cause skin sensitivity. Use caution when treating young children.

Lavender essential oil is known for its alcohols, ester, terpenes, phenols, oxides, and ketones. It is considered analgesic, anticoagulant, anti-convulsive, antidepressant, anti-fungal, antihistamine, anti-infectious, anti-inflammatory, antimicrobial, antimutagenic, antiseptic, antispasmodic, anti-toxic, anti-tumor, and used as a cardio tonic, regenerative, and sedative. Historically, it has been used for or as a calming agent, allergies, anxiety, appetite, arrhythmia, arteriosclerosis, bites/stings, blister, boils, breast tenderness, burns, cancer, chickenpox, concentration, convulsions, cuts, dandruff, depression, diaper rash, diuretic, dysmenorrhea, exhaustion, fever, gangrene, intestinal gas, grief, hay fever, herpes, hyperactivity, inflammation, insomnia, itching, mastitis, menopause, mental stress, mood swings, mosquito repellent, pain, poison ivy, rheumatoid arthritis, sedative, seizure, skin disorders, stretch marks, sunburn, tachycardia, teething pain, thrush, ticks ulcers, varicose veins, vertigo, worms, wounds and wrinkles. It can be used aromatically, topically, and orally.

Lemon essential oil is known for its terpenes, aldehydes, esters, and phenols. It is considered anticancer, antidepressant, antiseptic, anti-fungal, antioxidant, antiviral, astringent, invigorating, refreshing, and tonic. Historically, it has been used for anxiety, atherosclerosis, bites/stings, blood pressure, brain injury, cold sores, concentration, constipation, depression, digestion, disinfectant, dry throat, dysentery, energizer, exhaustion, fever, flu, furniture polish, gout, oily hair, grief, hangovers, heartburn, intestinal parasites, kidney stones, detox, overeating, pancreatitis, energy, relaxation, stress, sore throat, tonsillitis, varicose veins, and water purification. It can be used aromatically, topically, and orally. Topical use can cause sun sensitivity.

Tea tree essential oil is known for its terpenes, oxides, and alcohols. It is considered an analgesic, antibacterial, anti-fungal, anti-infectious, anti-inflammatory, antioxidant, antiparasitic, antiseptic, antiviral, decongestant, digestive, expectorant, immune stimulant, insecticidal, neurotoxic, stimulant, and tissue regenerative. Historically, it has been used for acne, allergies, aneurysm, athlete's foot, bacterial infections, boils, bronchitis, candida, canker sores, cavities, chickenpox, cold sores, colds, coughs, cuts, eczema, dry/itchy eyes, ear infections, flu, fungal infections, gum disease, hepatitis, hives, immunity boosting, wounds, infection, inflammation, lice, mumps, pink eye, rashes, ringworm, rubella, scabies, shingles, shock, sore throat, staph infections, sunburn, thrush, tonsillitis, viral infections, warts, and wounds. It can be used aromatically, topically and orally. Continued topical use can cause skin sensitivity.

Myrrh (as brought to Mary and Joseph) essential oil is known for its terpenes, furanoids, ketones, and phenols. It is considered anti-infectious, anti-inflammatory, antiseptic, anti-tumor, astringent, and tonic. Historically, it has been used for cancer, chapped skin, congestion, dysentery, gum disease, Hashimoto's, hepatitis, hypothyroidism, infection, liver cirrhosis, skin ulcer, stretch marks, and weeping wounds. It can be used aromatically, topically, and orally. Caution should be used during pregnancy.

Peppermint essential oil is known for its phenol alcohols, ketones, terpenes, esters, oxides, and phenols. It is considered analgesic, antibacterial, anti-carcinogenic, anti-inflammatory, antiseptic, antispasmodic, antiviral, and invigorating. Historically, it has been used for alertness, antioxidant, asthma, autism, bacterial infections, Bell's palsy, brain injury, fatigue, cold sores, colon polyps, congestion, constipation, cooling, cramps, Crohn's, diarrhea, dysmenorrhea, endurance, fainting, fever, flue, radiation exposure, gastritis, bad breath, headaches, heartburn, heatstroke, hernia, herpes, hives, hot flashes, hypothyroidism, indigestion, irritable bowel syndrome, itching, memory, migraines, motion sickness, multiple sclerosis, sore/tired muscles, nausea, loss of smell, osteoporosis, scabies, sciatica, shock, sinusitis, sore throat, typhoid, varicose veins, and vomiting. It can be used aromatically, topically, and orally. Repeated topical use can cause skin sensitivity. It can raise blood pressure. Use with caution during pregnancy.

Rosemary essential oil is known for its oxides, terpenes, ketones, alcohols, and phenols. It is considered analgesic, antibacterial, anticancer, anti-catarrhal, antifungal, anti-infectious, anti-inflammatory, antioxidant, and expectorant. Historically, it has been used for alcohol addiction, arterial vasodilator, arthritis, Bell's palsy, cancer, cellulite, chemical stress, cholera, constipation, detoxification, diabetes, diuretic, fainting, fatigue, flue, hair loss, headaches, inflammation, kidney infection, lice, low blood pressure, memory, osteoarthritis, sinusitis, vaginal infection, viral hepatitis, and worms. It can be used aromatically, topically, and orally. It is not for use during pregnancy or by people with epilepsy. It will raise blood pressure.

These are some examples of essential oils and their uses. There are many more essential oils and uses. Blending different essential oils together enhances certain aspects of each oil, creating a particular use for the blend. Not all oils or brands of oils are safe for consumption. Always use caution with essential oils.

Chapter 13

Can't I Ever Have Any Fun?

> These things I have spoken to you, that My joy may
> be in you, and that your joy may be made full.
>
> —John 15:11

Our culture equates having fun with things that are not always the best for us. Think of a birthday party. Many people don't think of fixing a gourmet meal to celebrate a birthday; they think of cake and ice cream. When we are truly eating God's way, we will find that man's foods just don't taste as good as they used to. But that doesn't mean we can't occasionally have a small amount of them.

Remember that we decided to eat God's way to be the best that we can be in our natural bodies. It has nothing to do with our spirituality. This means that when we want to indulge in a little bit of man's food, we can. Is it going to hurt us? Yes. Most of the times we find that we don't feel our best when we go back to eating man's way after eating God's way for a while. Will it be harder to eat God's way afterwards? Yes. Man's foods contain chemicals that are addicting. They feed the bacteria and cancer that is always in our systems. Going back and forth will be hard on your body. You will begin to forget how good it felt to truly eat God's way. The more you stray, the harder it will be to get back on the right path.

Isn't this the way it is with sin in our lives? We commit a small sin and we feel remorseful and vow never to do it again. Then another opportunity comes along and we find it easier to give in the second and third time. Before long, we are doing things we wouldn't have dreamed of doing before that first slip up. Eating can be the same way. The more we do it, the stronger the pull of the artificial foods.

When would we consider eating man's way? When we are invited to someone's house to eat and don't want to hurt feelings. God values relationships more than He values the physical body. Our bodies can handle the occasional poor food choices, where most relationships are much more fragile. When you eat at someone's house, eat the foods that are put before you and enjoy them. When they come to your house, show them just how good God's foods can really be.

Another time to relax your eating habits is when you are traveling. If you can't prepare all your food yourself, then make the best choices from what is available. Then don't fret about it. Restaurant food will rarely be God's food. Just do the best you can. When you get home, do some things to help your body clean itself and get back to Godly eating habits as soon as you can.

Chapter 14

But That's My Favorite Food!

Watch and pray that you may not enter into temptation;
the spirit indeed is willing, but the flesh is weak.

—Matthew 26:41

We all have a favorite food. It is usually something that is wrapped in strong childhood memories. Many times when you have been eating God's way and you get the opportunity to have that favorite food you find that it just doesn't taste as good as you remember. Other times it simply takes you back to those good memories, and you don't really care. There are a couple of ways to handle the favorite food dilemma.

The first is to try to make it at home using wholesome ingredients. Let's take an example of brownies. A package of brownie mix has all sorts of sugar and chemicals in it. It is definitely man's food and not God's. But there are many recipes from the paleo movement that show you how to make something that tastes just as good, or better, than that brownie mix. You can substitute coconut flour for the wheat flour. You can substitute honey for the sugar. Sometimes it will take a bit of trial and error to find out what satisfies your taste buds. Just make sure you are using whole foods instead of fake foods or chemicals.

For some of us, this concept backfires. Having something that tastes almost like what we remember makes us want that favorite food in its original form even more. For us, it is better to go cold turkey. Stay away from that food as much as possible. Using the example of the brownies, you may tell yourself that you will only indulge in them on your birthday. That way you are not telling yourself you can't have it, you are just limiting when you will indulge in it.

Chapter 15

Fasting

> Whenever you fast, do not put on a gloomy face as they hypocrites do, for they neglect their appearance so that they will be noticed by men when they are fasting. Truly I say to you, they have their reward in full.
>
> —Matthew 6:16

The Bible talks about fasting. It talks about it helping you to become closer with God. This closeness is on an emotional and spiritual level. Just by breaking habits and changing routines, you can become more aware of your world and the role God plays in it. Fasting goes much deeper than that.

Fasting changes the way your body behaves. Going without food for a period of time triggers the body to begin a cleaning phase. It doesn't take as long as you would think to start this process. The longer the fast lasts, the deeper the cleansing goes.

Twenty years ago, our experts were telling us that we needed to eat three to six times a day. Their theory was that if you never get hungry then you won't be tempted to overeat or eat the wrong foods. That actually works for some people. For others, life becomes one continuing binge. The more they eat, the worse their choices become. Eating this often sets your body up to burn sugars (carbohydrates).

When you skip or delay the first meal of the day, your body thinks you are beginning a fast. It has already gone all night without eating and it is primed to go into the cleansing mode. This mode sets you up to burn fats. This is in preparation for breaking down the body's own fat supplies to sustain it until food is available again. God designed our bodies this way so that we can endure times when food was scarce, such as droughts and long winters.

This delay of foods is called intermittent fasting. If you are in general good health and you want to ensure your body is at peak operation, intermittent fasting may be exactly what you are looking for. It will rev up your metabolism and teach your body to burn fats instead of carbohydrates. Fats take longer to burn, and we store the excess within the body so it is always available. Once you are used to the difference, you will find that you function better when your body is in fat-burning mode.

Before the advent of modern medicine, many illnesses were treated with fasting. When we are ill, the body naturally shuts down the digestive system.

Early man didn't eat if they weren't hungry. Instead, they drank pure water to keep themselves hydrated and sometimes other liquids such as clear bone broth. This kept the body hydrated without needing to use energy for digestion. Instead, the body used all available energy to clean the body from the inside out. The concept still works today.

Many illnesses can be avoided, or even cured, by cleansing the body internally. Fasting is one of the ways to do this.

Juice fasting is a modified form of fasting. With juice fasting, you are supplementing your fast with the fresh juice only of fruits and/or vegetables. This gives your body access to the vitamins and minerals that it doesn't have in storage. Juice fasting only really works with freshly juiced fruits and vegetables. Even if you could get preserved fruit and vegetable juices without a lot of sugars and additives, they still would not work as well as the ones you freshly juice each time you want them. The reason is that the vitamins and minerals you are seeking the most are the ones that disappear the fastest once the food is broken down by the process of extracting the juice. You can get almost the same effect with simply pureeing the fresh vegetables. The more ill you are, the purer your juice needs to be.

CHAPTER 16

WHAT ABOUT THE PEOPLE AROUND ME?

> Therefore let no one act as your judge in regard to food
> or drink or in respect to a festival or a new moon or a
> Sabbath day—things which are a mere shadow of what
> is to come; but the substance belongs to Christ.
>
> —Colossians 2:16

Judge not that ye shall not be judged, or at least something along that line. When we find something that really makes us feel better, whether it is physically or emotionally, we want to share it with everyone around us. This is what we did when we first accepted Christ as our Savior. It will also be a tendency when you begin eating God's way. Just as everybody did not automatically accepted Christ for themselves on your word alone, they are not going to start eating God's way on your word alone. They may never decide to eat God's way. Even otherwise strong Christians do not always understand that the way we eat is part of giving

God a living sacrifice of our lives. When this happens you just have to love them anyway.

On one hand, I noticed it the most when eating at restaurants. It used to drive me crazy when I would see what family members ordered. I would want to explain to them again what chemicals were in those foods and why they shouldn't be eating them. Then I realized that wasn't my place. I had not been put on this earth to judge them. I started putting on mental blinders whenever I went to a restaurant or a pot luck dinner. I would make the best choices for myself and try my hardest not to notice what others around me were eating. When I can do it, it takes the anxiety out of the meal.

On the other hand, once you have tried to explain this concept of eating, people are going to be looking at what is on your plate. I have run into friends at restaurants, and they don't try to hide the fact that they are checking out my plate. They want to see if I practice what I preach. It is even worse at pot luck dinners. Sometimes at pot lucks, the choice is to make poor choices or go hungry. I always try to bring something healthy to eat and load up my plate with that. Then I will take a little bit of some other dishes that don't look too bad. People watch me in line and on the way back to my table. They also come over to chat while I am eating. I am sure it is really to check out what I am eating. Remember, just like the world is watching you to see if you are acting like a Christian, when others know that you are trying to eat God's way, they will be watching that as well.

Chapter 17

Your Mouth Isn't the Only Thing That Eats

For no one ever hated his own flesh, but nourishes and cherishes it, just as Christ also does the church.

—Ephesians 5:29

We have talked a lot about what you put in your mouth and why. Now we want to talk about how else things get into your body, both good and bad things.

You have heard that your skin is the largest organ of the body. When we think about the skin, we usually think of it as a protective shield around our body. In some ways it is, but that isn't all it does. Our skin is also one of the ways we get rid of toxins. When we sweat, toxins in the body are pushed out the sweat glands along with the moisture. Sweat cools the body, but it also gets rid of junk that we have put in the body. We have all been around people that as they sweat you pick up on a strong odor. It may be garlic, cigarette smoke, or, if they have been exposed to it, some chemical. Our lymph system is intimately paired with our sweat system. They work together to get rid of stuff. When we inhibit the sweat system from working properly, we inhibit our bodies from detoxification.

Chemical antiperspirants are a good example. They control the moisture through closing or blocking the sweat glands so moisture cannot escape. The toxins that are ready and waiting to be dumped through the moisture then back up into the surrounding tissue. It is highly probable that this is one of the causes of breast cancer. Since those toxins cannot be released, it is surmised that they back up into the milk production glands. These glands highly resemble the sweat glands but with a different purpose.

Unfortunately, the skin also acts as a two-way valve. If you think of a damp sponge, you will get the idea. Sweating is like squeezing out the sponge. When you let go of the sponge, it will then absorb anything (in this case liquid) that it comes in contact with. This can be good or bad.

To demonstrate this, try cutting garlic clove in half and rubbing the cut side on the underside of your foot. Try to count how long it takes before you taste garlic. For most people, it is only a second or two. Have you ever gone swimming and even after a shower you smell like chlorine? This is because you skin has absorbed the chlorine from the pool water.

You can utilize this aspect of the human body for your benefit. An Epsom salt bath works in two ways. The sodium in the Epsom salts will draw impurities (toxins) from your body into the water. At the same time, the magnesium in the Epsom salts will be absorbed into the body. Many supplements can be used this way. The most common are coconut oil and magnesium. Both go in through the skin and nourish the body.

The same action can also put you in danger. Putting chemicals on the skin allows the skin to absorb those chemicals. People think nothing of rubbing a chemical-laden hand lotion or perfume on their skin, but the body is not designed to get rid of chemicals. Shampoos, conditioners, hair spray, hair coloring, and other such products are absorbed into the skin of the scalp, and from there, into the brain. Some things are stopped by the blood-brain barrier, but not everything.

The other way we take in toxins and nutrients is through our lungs. Every time we breathe, we both take in and get rid of stuff. This is one reason why aromatherapy works. We breathe in the small partials of essential oils. Unfortunately, we also breathe in small particles of petroleum products and other chemicals. We can't eliminate all of them, but we can reduce our toxic load by eliminating the ones we can.

In the home, cleaning products and air fresheners are the major culprits. More and more we have cleaner options to replace these chemical products. Outdoors, it is chemical pesticides, fertilizers, and the like. If the neighboring farmer is spraying his fields, you aren't going to be able to stop him, but you can go inside and close the windows until he is done.

Chapter 18

What Are the Results?

> The wicked earns deceptive wages, but he who
> sows righteousness gets a true reward.
>
> —Proverbs 11:18

The result of choosing properly grown food and preparing them in a variety of ways is a life full of adventure. This adventure is not just in the kitchen or around the dining table but in all of life. A diet consisting of a rainbow of vibrant, natural colors will lead to a vibrant outlook on life. It also has a tendency to lead to other areas of our lives where we wish to follow God. These might include our internal lives, social lives, our physical fitness, and in the products that we use on our hair and skin as well as throughout our homes.

When we take control of our health, our internal lives tend to change. Instead of blaming genetics, the environment, the government, or even our parents for our problems, we begin taking personal responsibility. When we feel better about ourselves, we can also begin looking beyond ourselves and seeing the needs of others. Sometimes we even have the energy to help someone else.

Our social lives also begin to change. Instead of revolving around processed foods, we enjoy spending time with others creating really good food. We also look beyond food for entertainment. This can mean more time interacting with others.

Since we have more energy, we can look for new ways to use that energy. This can be done while socializing or in a more prescribed method many of us refer to as exercise. It can also lead to doing more things for yourself that you used to pay others to do. This often means more projects in and around the house. This, in turn, can lead to saving more money that would have been spent on what we are now making for ourselves.

Once we realize the harm that chemicals in and on our food have on our bodies, we often begin looking for the other sources of chemicals in our lives. This might mean replacing chemical air fresheners with essential oils or organic potpourri. It could also mean replacing chemical shampoos, conditioners, and other hair products with more natural ones. Many women decide to go to natural makeup or give up makeup altogether. Natural deodorants work well when you realize that the chemical antiperspirants are one of the causes of cancer. There are many aspects of our lives that we can clean up and begin doing it God's way, but that can be another book.

Conclusion

The conclusion, when all has been heard, is: fear God and keep His commandments, because this applies to every person.

—Ecclesiastes 12:13

God honors us when we honor Him. This doesn't mean that when we start eating His way all of our troubles will go away. Satan is going to find a way to attack. There is no doubt about that. What it does mean is that as we are going about our lives, trying to be transformed into His image, more things will seem to go right for us. Even the things that don't go right will somehow be easier for us to handle. Earlier I spoke about our emotions being on a more even-keel. This is something that I have seen happen time and time again as people change their eating habits.

Depression disappears. You are more able to see the joy and beauty in life than you did eating man's way. This is because the chemicals in the food are not dragging you down. Low blood sugar is also not dragging you down.

Illness disappears, or at least improves. God designed us to be self-healing, but we have to have the body's building blocks available for the body to do so. God also designed us to be self-cleaning. If we limit the garbage we put into our body through our mouth, lungs, and skin, our body will be able to clean up from the stress of day to day living. If we put in more garbage than our body can hold, it becomes like an overflowing trash can. We call the results illness.

Changing habits never comes easy. Completely changing your lifestyle is even harder. Taking one day at a time makes it a little more manageable. Strive today to live a little cleaner than yesterday. Each time you go to the store, try not to bring any more garbage home. Eventually, you will look around and see that you are living a fairly clean life.

Printed in the United States
By Bookmasters